RIDE A WAVE

Anastasia Turner

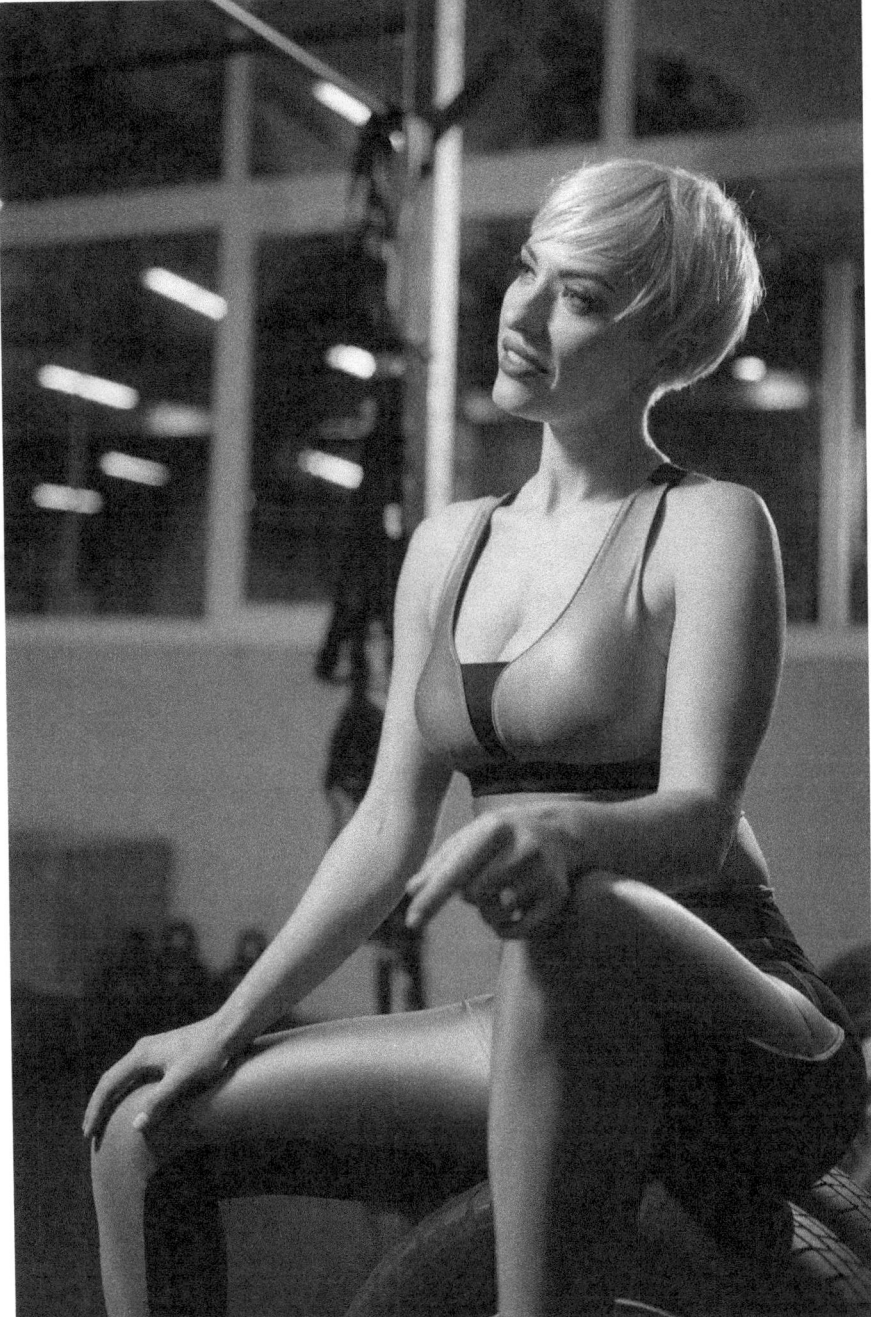

A fit-hit for losing weight!

Ride a wave!

Motivation right from the start!

The true story of a plum girl's makeover into a super-woman

This book is for the girls and women who are eager to have a thin body and gain self-confidence and independence. Get a chance to reverse course and change your life for the better by using Anastasia's real life example.

The main character is going to reveal the secrets and tell you how to achieve major weight loss, allowing you to live out your dream and become a better version of yourself.

You can do it!

CONTENTS

Preface

If I ever had the opportunity of writing a letter about my past, I wouldn't be very wordy.

"Anastasia, stop eating too much! Your life depends on it!"

It was difficult for me to overcome my strong addiction to food, and because of it, I went down a long, complicated path towards recovery. But now I want to share my story with you so you won't have to go down that same dark path.

Needless to say, I am proud of the results I achieved and I am more than happy with the woman I became.

But first, let me warn you. My story is not about some special magical cure-all. There won't be no-effort stories of the fat on my belly melting away into nothingness if I'm chowing down on 10 hamburgers a day. This book is my life story regarding my change from a plumper to a slender lady.

Let's roll!

Here is your FREE gift! Follow this link http://e-book.tilda.ws/rideawave1 and you will get a bunch of my great photos!

Introduction

"The only way to lose weight is to restore purpose to life,"
- Cyril Connolly

I used to be an ordinary child with fairly normal body composition and I didn't really care much about my body and appearance.

I was fond of chicken wings, burgers, and pizza and the major part of my diet was loaded with calories, greasy, and usually extremely sweet or spicy. It was, without a doubt, delicious. For dinner, my menu consisted of prepackaged food, potato chips, or French fries in some golden-colored cheese sauce. It was so cozy sitting in front of my computer screen in my favorite fluffy pajamas, eating junk food and watching TV shows. Time just flew by, filled with overwrought angst and colorful emotions, but the food on my plate disappeared even faster, like in magician's trick. Poof! My plate would be empty! When something extremely exciting was happening on the screen, I surely would want extra food, so my empty plate would be full again almost instantly.

In the morning, my mom always humored me with a delicious breakfast. I remember that I didn't like getting up for school, but the attractive fragrance from the kitchen did a great job of kicking me out of bed! Barefooted, I would shoot out of bed and would be seated at the table dressed, washed, and even with my hair done. The table would be filled with my favorite doughnuts and hot chocolate, homemade cookies, fruits, pudding, peanut butter pie, brownies, muffins, cheesecakes, you name it. A variety of my breakfast consisted of so many scrumptious things that one could publish a cookbook with all the picturesque sweets that were there.

At school, I used to have pizza of a hamburger for lunch followed by a sweet yogurt or juice. It was quick and satisfying! Imagine a schoolgirl stuffing her face with chocolate doughnuts, then the tardy bell rings! I would be running late to the class while chewing quickly. Thanks to my mum, who always put wet tissues in my backpack otherwise, my hands would be so sticky.

Teachers taught us all about spelling, math, science, and how to find the square root of 64, but they did forget one thing. Teachers forgot to give us the skills we need to be healthy. They didn't teach us how to watch our weight.

In high school, I didn't lose my habit of eating honey buns during break. Somewhere deep inside, I desired to get rid of it, but it was not easy - the journey of no return was already embarked upon. You can clearly imagine how buns affected my appearance. The first sign of my close friendship with pastries was already easy to be seen. My hip pouring over my belt happened to be the biggest issue for me.

At that time, I had sleep disorders, which made me irritable and prompted me into watching films late into the night. I didn't realize that gluttony was responsible for such a strong dependence, leading me not only to various digestive diseases, but also body malfunctioning as a whole. Such a condition threatened my body with irreversible consequences along with psychological disorders. I was impulsive, emotionally unstable, and doing sudden and unpredictable things.

When food is abused, eating is like a narcotic leading to a full-blown addiction. This was something I started to realize gradually. Understanding my abuse generated guilt and depression. I was eating while being nervous and I was then anxious about gluttony. Somewhere deep in my subconscious, I understood that something was wrong, but my habit overpowered my better judgment. It was comfortable to follow the unhealthy habits I've made, I felt cozy and peaceful.

Careless and irrational behavior about my appearance would not last long. When I was 14, I fell in love with my classmate, a handsome, sweet guy. He was tall, slim, athletic, with dimples on his cheeks. He would even play with his hair while talking to me! Every single girl in our class liked him.

You would think that I was part of such "competition." Well, actually I wasn't deprived of beauty. I highly valued myself, felt myself to be easy-going and loose. I was a funny, confident and trendy girl, and I always had enough of boys' attention. Needless to say, the crush was mutual, despite the fact that I was an obese girl.

I think every girl remembers those first, naïve feelings when you can do anything for love... well, almost anything. I was extremely eager to look slimmer and every inch attractive - I finally understood that I had to do something! But breaking up with buns was much harder than I expected!

Overcoming fear, for the first time in my life, I started taking part in sports. There were 20 people in my team, only two of us were girls.

I hated workouts. Each time we were all running, practicing and playing on the field, I had only one thought: "When will I finally go home and eat something tasty?" I was dreaming to have washboard stomach, but it had other plans and hid somewhere far under the layer of fat on my belly.

I, a teenage girl, didn't understand the simple rules of a gym life. Closed-toed shoes, sneakers, two towels — one for the shower and the other for workouts. I was too shy to ask the trainer any questions and everything was new and unusual, even the names - disks, bars, dumbbells. What the heck are those? I had to learn how to use the tools, where to put them, how to do the basic exercise set. How could I possibly know that stepping over the bar when an athlete wants to lift it is rude? In short, I was an awkward stranger in a strange land.

My enthusiasm disappeared quickly and the guys from the gym added fuel to the fire. Those "musclemen" covered with tattoos, having chains on their pumped-up necks, with the bared teeth of predators on their T-shirts began throwing insults about my round forms, especially one mountain of meat who had a hideous, scraggly red beard. He constantly made it his mission to hurt me. Of course, these "jokes" might just be rude flirts, but it was very painful and hurt so bad for me to hear "fritter, gingerbread, and doughnut" and similar nicknames aimed at me. These guys were adults, I couldn't answer them in any way and I suffered through it all. I felt depressed. Terrible, anxious thoughts filled my mind, plunging me into a deep depression. To crawl out of this nightmare, I was even more tempted by junk food, which naturally led to more weight gain. So, I abandoned sports quickly, but now, in addition to being overweight, I was also screwed-up. I looked at myself in the mirror, yearned, and dreamed of a chic figure, a stunning sexy appearance filled with charm and charisma.

Having resigned myself to the idea that doing sports is not for me, I threw in the towel. And the fatter I grew, the darker my horizon was. I stopped dreaming of a beautiful future for myself and started doing things to keep me busy. I learned how to play computer games, I started drawing, I went to the park for walks, and I even got two cats (as they are proven partners of female solitude).

I also became eager to bake pastries – I painted gingerbread cookies, I cooked cupcakes and cakes. And I kept on winding my way through life with my plump feet.

From time to time, a light bulb turned on in my mind – I started maintaining a healthy diet, I tried exercising at home (because I didn't have the courage to go back to the gym), and I jogged outside. I even managed to lose several pounds. It was an incredible victory for me. You can't even imagine how proud I was!

But my family and friends didn't support me in my goal to lose weight. Mum thought I was after the fashionable trends and beauty standards and she'd always say something like:

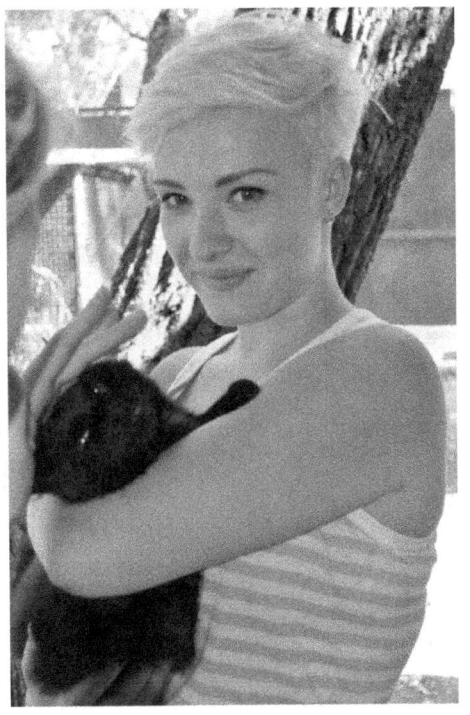

"Anastasia, why are you troubling yourself with this? You're a very beautiful girl! Don't be silly, you don't need to lose weight. This modern trend of being thin doesn't cater to an individual's constitution. You need to love yourself and your appearance as it is otherwise, you'll spend life chasing those unattainable beauty trends."

Such phrases disillusioned me and I went back to regular life with my best friends – junk food, pizza, and hamburgers.

My life was a continuous and absolute fight. One part of me strived to have a flat belly, slim thighs, and a thin waist. The other part of my personality, however, would prefer eating candy, no matter what.

At 22, I found a good vacant position at an advertising agency and from the very beginning, I liked the atmosphere and tone at the office. Communication with interesting people gave me the possibility to learn a lot. A good salary satisfied my funding needs and I got to participate in creative projects to feed my artistic ambitions. I've learned everything very quickly: how to print documents, process orders, and communicate with clients. Company policy was rather democratic – the working atmosphere was very friendly and we also had retreat parties, we went camping to relax, chill out, and cope with stress because we often stayed at work late.

Gradually, stress started to emerge. I constantly lacked free time, the job was sedentary; I'd sit at the computer screen, and I had a lot of stress due to interpersonal relationships. Sometimes I'd go home after work without having eaten anything during the day. So, I'd order greasy takeout, stuff myself, and go to bed.

Joke

-Single women come home, see what's in the fridge, and go to bed. Married women come home, see what's in bed, and then go to the fridge.

In the morning, I'd go back to work. Office... home... office...home – this vicious circle continued for two years. I had no idea how it would all end at the time, but one important event did happen.

First, let me say that I never had scales at home. Why would I? I didn't need them. It was never my aim to buy them and then look at the number only to make myself depressed! It was clear to me that scales wouldn't make me happy.

One day, I went to the production facility to manage an extremely important cargo shipment for our client. It was a large room with scales and a pile of goods ready to be shipped after being weighed. While finishing up my work, I decided to weigh myself, just for the fun of it. I will never forget the number scales showed – 78 kilos. Then, I remembered I was only 165cm tall! A bolt of lightning hit me and everything that happened next was in a fog. I suddenly got the striking realization that I was fat! How could I have ignored it for so long?

I didn't remember my way home. I hardly could recognize things happening around me. I had only one thought, blinking in my brain: "I'm fat, I'm fat, I'm fat…"

I felt so tired that I simply passed out right when I got home. That day, I had nightmares – everybody was pointing at me, hissing at and saying cruel things like: "You're disgusting, you are ugly, you're horrible! Shame!" Monsters hunted me down only to scold me.

When I woke up the following morning, covered in clammy sweat, I had a rapid change of mind. Some unexplained and strange power was awaking within me. Without further ado, I clearly and openly recognized the matter of the heart. Now, I call it "riding the wave" like in the movie Surf's Up (from 2007).

So, I started an active campaign to completely meet my goal. I knew the result I was going to end up with. I had a flawless, precise image in my mind, as if someone had drawn it in my brain. I was playing the film in my head on a loop, inspired to set the Thames on fire. I had a visual image of self – slim, strong, strapped, and confident, making it my inner strength.

Chapter 1: Turning up the Heat!

"Dieting is the only game where you win when you lose!"
— *Karl Lagerfeld*

When making an action plan, I set objectives and took small steps towards victory. Every properly taken step fueled my confidence and inspired me to go further.

Here are some examples of my everyday routine:

During lunch, my colleagues ate all kinds of junk food, but I ate steamed broccoli and hard-boiled eggs. I salivated watching my coworkers eat, but I kept saying to myself: "Come on, Anastasia, stay strong. You can do it!" I heard dozens of jokes about my lunch! It was ok to hear it from my peers, but then my boss joined in...

Just to give you an idea – it was exactly like in the movie "Horrible Bosses".

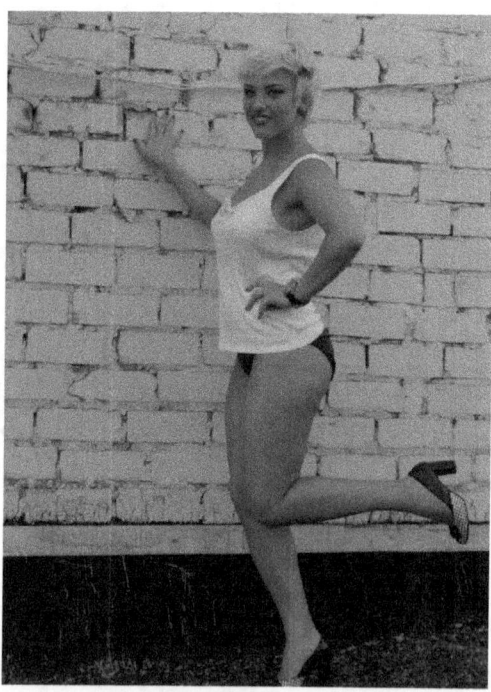

To keep up with my fitness plan, I jogged every day after work. My boss, who liked calling in the evening after work to... talk about work, demanded a complete report on my progress at work. I fruitlessly tried to explain that I am busy with an important thing right now and I can't chat. I needed to prioritize my time. Me, wearing a training suit, ready to go, but I couldn't! I even told my boss about my dream of becoming slim and fit. I shared my dream of getting rid of extra fat in my body and about the need to practice every day.

He just didn't want to hear it. And then, he started calling me after work even more often! He was eating up all of my free time with useless talk, as if he intended to distract me from training! He himself was far from being an athlete. Jugging ears, a flabby stomach, and glistening bare spots on his head made him especially unattractive. His shrilling voice didn't add any points to his charm as well.

On some occasions, I decided not to pick up, but then a shower of calls would find its way to my phone. Then he'd call my friend I was working together with. One day, after having seen 10 missed calls, my patience finally snapped. I picked up the ringing phone and exploded. There was a threatening silence on the other end of the line, I was predicting a storm over my head and over what was left of my career at the advertising firm. The dreams of my upward movement within the agency lay in ruins. I braced myself, waiting. I wanted to scream and cry, but I was silent and the silence that I got in response was the clearest possible answer.

At that moment I got it. "I need to quit!" I said to myself. Don't think for a moment that it was an easy decision. I loved my job. I was attracted to it, attracted to the lifestyle it offered, to the people, the workplace, my responsibilities, and my privileges. But what would you choose: Your health and private life or a job for a boss who had no respect for your goals?

In a month, I packed up and left. I said goodbye to everyone at the agency, and also to my weight. I opened a new door to an exciting world where I, slim and confident, am full of new hopes and perspectives.

The first thing I did was go to Belmar, my favorite resort town on the Atlantic shores of New Jersey. Imagine how I felt walking alone along the hot and humid streets. Swimming was prohibited at the time because of the strong waves coming in and the seagulls were walking together with me in search of something to snack on. I was surprised that the birds were afraid of nothing on the beach and that they didn't care they were fat.

I was driving along the town, viewing those small white houses, the clean streets, the perfect lawns, and all the people laying back and relaxing. Those new and bright emotions gave new birth to my hopes and dreams. I realized that I belonged here; I had, again, enough power and was ready to roll.

The "new me" came back home. It was like I washed

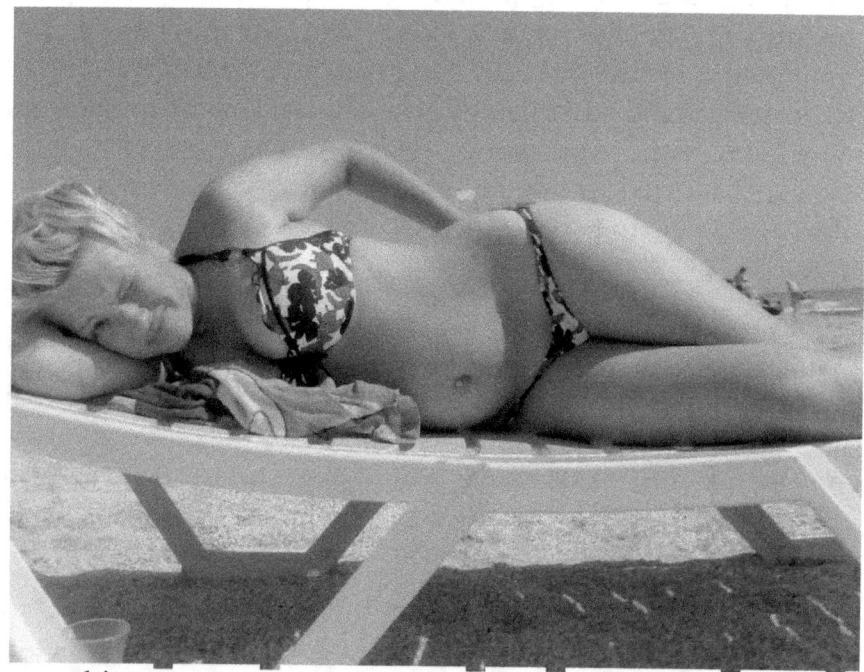

everything extra, unnecessary, and superficial away. I changed my life rapidly. I changed my schedule, my habits, and my mindset. I even remember my first time in a fitness class as though it was yesterday. I was shy stepping into that training room, wearing that horrible huge T-shirt to cover everything imperfect under it. The nice smile of the trainer girl and her tender voice empowered me. Her appearance and trimmed figure motivated me to practice even more.

I was jumping on steppers, did push-ups, squats, and trunk curls for four months. Rhythmic modern music, I was surrounded by a group of plump girls just like myself. We did sets together and trained, trained, trained. Finally, the scales deducted 8 kilos from my previous weight. Now, everybody around has started noticing the changes happening to me; not only in my appearance, but also the intrinsic changes.

My happy wave was taking me further into the future. You see, of course, I wanted immediate results. It was unbearable

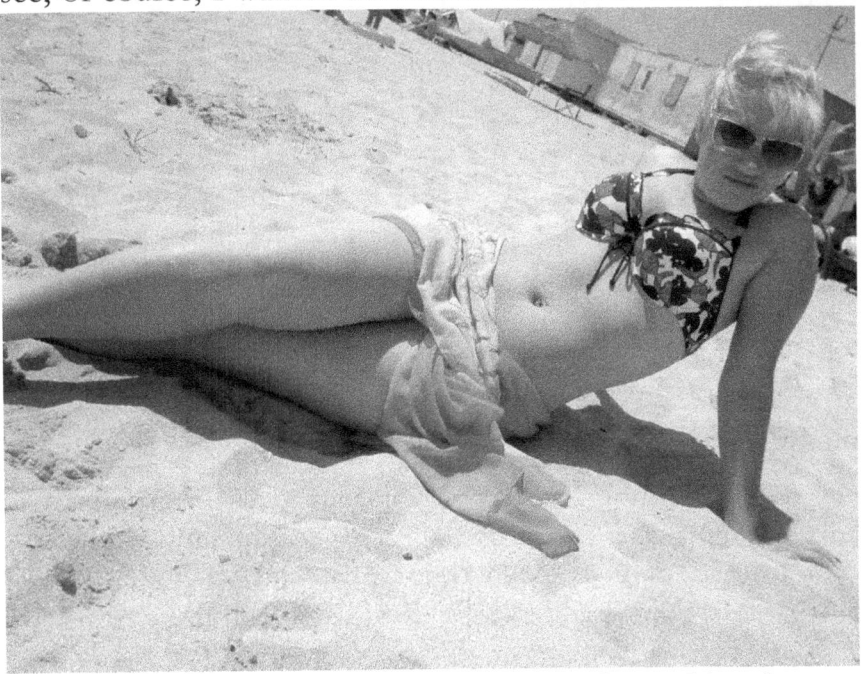

to be in that fat body. I kept searching and searching for new weight loss methods. Once, I even heard about the high-protein diet called "Maggie". My trainer tried to reason with me by warning that the lost weight will come back quickly. But I've already made my decision. I stocked up on eggs and chicken, as well as those separated containers for split meals. There was no going back!

The next month went by the predetermined schedule – I had a special time for every meal. I knew exactly what kind of breakfast, lunch, and dinner I would have. My menu had mostly meat, fish, eggs, veggies, fruits, cottage cheese, and – extremely rarely – cereal. That's it!

Was it easy? NO! But when you see your goal in front of you, no one can stop you.

My close relatives can bear witness to the hardship of sticking to such a strict dietary regime. At some point, they even tried to "reason" with me.

Once and again, nothing could stop me. I was an icebreaker, breaking through the ice like a sailor who strived to reach the sacred coast. I couldn't be stopped.

During the first month of my diet, I lost 7 kilos. The next month it was 6 kilos, and then I gained my self-confidence. 57 kilos of weight were the first serious accomplishment and true victory I had made for myself. I lost **21 kilos** in six months!

I heard compliments from people every day, I heard: "How could you possibly do it?" so often. My answer was simple: "Ride your wave!"

After six months of continuous training and self-improvement, I reached a point that impressed even me! I kept following the chosen training and eating plan. Today, my stable weight is 52-53 kilos. But don't think that my fight is over! No, I still want to eat chocolate bars and candy, and sometimes I want to allow myself time to relax, but in those cases, Socrates' words sound off in my head loud: "We're living not for eating, but eating for living."

Here, you are given the opportunity to use the same steps as I have so that you can be happy with how you look in the mirror. Using my own personal example, I will tell you how the methods work and the milestones you should avoid. Together, we'll find out what frequently made mistakes are waiting for you and what misrepresentations you will face when losing weight.

We'll talk about eating, sugar, and training. Those are the three pillars of my system. Three supporting bars.

The chapters of the book are designed to be separate – you can read the book in its entirety or you can pick up on any chapter separately. Look closely, read some passages aloud, feel the text, follow the reaction of your body and mind. How did you react to what you just read? Ask yourself, do you believe the author? Only after you start thinking these pieces of advice are for you - adopt the information written here in this book.

This book is written as a guide, but I tried to make it fun and interesting for you. A whole team was dedicated to working out the material, united by one great idea: "You can become better and make your life awesome!"

We'll try to overcome fears, doubts, inertia, and the resistance from the environment together. The tools you've already tried do not work. All those goji berries, pills, bracelets, slimming teas, dietary supplements, super diets, endless weighing of yourself, fat-burning activators, metabolic regulators – did any of those lead to weight loss? I thought not.

And if you really need to lose weight, become slim, attractive, toned, and sexy, we need to act right now! In each part of the book, you'll find not only specific practical advice for you, but also motivational aphorisms, attitudes, and I hope we will go this way together joyfully, cheerfully, and effectively. Good luck!

Chapter 2: Diet – A Sensible Approach

There are only two ways:
Be happy with stuffing, or be happy with your reflection
in the mirror.

Before following diet recommendations, I recommend useful **Secret #1**.

Using only this tip, you can achieve your goal – weight loss.

Zip the belt over the protruding part of your stomach. Make it tight, but it shouldn't restrict breathing. Tightening the waist creates pressure onto the stomach reducing its volume. Using a belt for two weeks reduces a stomach and, consequently, prevents you from eating too much. Now, with the new stomach size it is easy to size your meal: put your palms cup together. This is a healthy measure for one meal. Actually, you can stop reading now – you reached the final goal – eating less.

"Neither satiety nor hunger, neither any other thing which shall exceed the measure of nature, can be good or healthful,"
- Hippocrates

"I am a better person when I have less on my plate,"
— Elizabeth Gilbert (Eat, Pray, Love)

Let's list the most common mistakes people make when losing weight:

✓ A sharp transition to low-calorie, low fat, low nutritional-content foods.
✓ Reducing the meal number by prolonging "fastening" in between them.
✓ Refusal to eat after 6 p.m.
✓ Dinner is the highest-calorie meal.
✓ Improper drinking regimen.
✓ Intake of carbohydrates and fatty foods.

So, my personal approach to nutrition is this:

My morning begins with a glass of lemon water on an empty stomach.

I think that most people have heard about the stunning effects that this has on the body, but for some strange reason people neglect it.

Just one glass of room-temperature water in the morning will help us:

- Lose weight.
- Wash out the toxins from our body.
- Preserve our youth.
- Start the metabolic process in the body.
- Send a message to our brain that it's time to start a new day.

Drinking water in the morning is a must! During the night, the body loses fluid and its level needs to be restored. Water is the perfect solvent for removing toxins. It cleanses everything - the blood, lymph, which, in turn, will improve the state of the skin, strengthen our hair, nails, and bones, and create the base for muscle strength. The work of the heart is facilitated as the body's endurance influences all the systems and organs to work efficiently. A simple drink of water on an empty stomach sets a new level of productivity, and you will immediately glow with health from the inside.

Lemon juice diluted with water is less aggressive than the fruit alone. Lemon water turns out into a balanced cocktail containing macro and micro elements and vitamins, thus anti-oxidizing the body. And more importantly, it limits the flow of glucose into the blood. Lemon water normalizes the excretory function of the intestines, helps in breaking down complex fat molecules and the alkaline blood balance normalizes. The benefits of lemon water are near infinite. But don't drink it if:

- You have a disease of the gastrointestinal tract (gastritis, ulcer, etc.), especially when in a relapse. We warn people with high stomach acidity: the intake of the drink on an empty stomach can lead to pain in the abdomen!

- You have a kidney disease. B vitamins that are part of citric acid have a strong diuretic effect. On the other hand, they contribute to the removal of kidney stones, but it can cause severe and unbearable pain.
- You have sensitive teeth. Citric acid can cause pain in the mouth, because its regular use makes enamel thinner. But using a straw to drink it can help.

Like in any field, use common sense, be cautious, and know when to stop. Do not over exaggerate or calm down your enthusiasm! Listen to your body's reaction; feel the changes and reactions and determine your opinion. And remember, everything will be okay!

If you don't have any of the above health issues, you can confidently drink a glass of water. Feel free to add lemon juice in the amount that is right for you. Welcome to the club of healthy people!

You can eat 15-30 minutes after a drink.

One of the most common mistakes when losing weight is to skip breakfast or make it as small as possible. Do not skip breakfast! Otherwise, you will definitely stuff yourself throughout the day.

Here lies the important weight-loss **Secret #2**.

Breakfast should be the highest-calorie meal of the day.

Breakfast is meant to supply the body with the energy it will need for the whole day. It should be rich with color and have an aesthetic pleasure. It is necessary to feed all the senses - sight, hearing, taste, smell, and the tactile receptors of the tongue and fingertips, to please both the body and the soul.

The food must be freshly prepared, healthy, and blessed.

Do not limit yourself with a cup of coffee for breakfast – it's not food, but cheating.

Secret #3

My perfect breakfast is eggs!

Eggs contain healthy protein that allows you to maintain a feeling of being full for longer.

No, wait, don't be so happy! It's not about fried eggs, fried in grease with bacon or sausage. Sorry, but it's better to cook an omelet with vegetables (tomatoes, bell peppers, spinach) or cook hard-boiled or poached eggs.

All sorts of green stuff go well with eggs too. Broccoli, zucchini, spinach, asparagus, green beans, squash, green peas, and other herbs, which will satisfy the body's daily need of vitamins and minerals.

Secret #4

As mentioned above, we should try to include the largest possible variety of food colors - yellow, red, green peppers, purple cabbage, purple eggplant, etc. The principle is clear. We delight the eye and we saturate the body with health and begin our day with vibrant creativity. The food we eat must be fit for a queen.

When choosing products for salads, consider their taste compatibility. Sour juices, berries, and fruits can be added to all vegetable and leaf salads. Sour fruits often improve the taste of vegetables.

Use new combinations and products every day. One high-protein product - fish, cottage cheese, low-fat turkey, chicken, beans, legumes, or peas. Just combine any meal with a fresh vegetable salad.

Secret #5

Having one piece of protein food (meat, fish, etc.) makes a portion of the vegetable salad being two times bigger than the protein component , which is especially true for green veggies.

One hour after a tasty and hearty breakfast, you can drink a glass of grapefruit juice.

Chapter 3: No Sugar

When reading the Chupa-Chups candy ingredients, you realize that it's better to eat the stick to stay healthy.

Secret #6

If you want to have a beautiful body, first you need to stop eating sweets: sugar, pastries, candies, chocolate, cakes, cookies, and other sweet delicacies. The same goes for carbonated drinks: Pepsi, Cola, Fanta, and sweet juices. Get rid of dairy-sweetened products - yogurt, cheese, mousses, and desserts. Your position must be unambiguous.

Joke

The box said it was 2 pounds of chocolate. So why did I gain 10 pounds?

"Inside every fat girl is a thin girl trying to get out,"
- Terry Pratchett

I recommend you to watch documentaries about sugar in order to fully understand and "know" the enemy backwards and forwards. That way you have a better idea of how to fight it and what to expect from it.

That Sugar Film, 2014

Director Damon Gamo shot an experiment on camera, during which the whole truth about sugar comes out. Almost all of our "healthy" food contains sugar. A highly professional documentary, it is both interesting and instructive to watch. The conclusions are unambiguous. After watching this movie, your life will never be the same.

Jamie's Sugar Rush

Here, the director is studying a variety of sugar additives used to create the food we eat. Research confirms that sugar negatively affects the human body.

Fed Up

This film is about how the food industry makes a lot of money from ordinary consumers, luring us with ad slogans and promises of health benefits for products that are completely opposite. Food is not what it used to be. Chemical technologies and genetic engineering have become firmly established in our lives, having introduced GMOs, food additives, flavor enhancers, dyes, preservatives, bleaches, baking powder, and other substitutes for ordinary, healthy food. The film seriously makes us think what we stuff into our bodies is unhealthy. After all, we are what we eat.

So it is better to start the major body cleansing of the *white drug* only after having watched the above films.

"When a person is upset, he eats candies...
Probably, they are plugging holes.
The boy finally understood why candies in boxes are round, square, and triangular.
Just no one knows in advance what form his sad hole will be..."
- Nadeya Yasminska

What do you call a sad coffee?

Depresso.

And so, here is the list of the harmful products that you are better off giving up:

- Sugar, sweeteners, and all products that contain sugar.
- Sweet drinks and alcohol (cola, lemonade, juice).
- Pastries (white bread, buns, puff pastry).
- Mayonnaise, sauces, burgers, hot dogs, and junk food.
- Confectionery (sweets, cookies, chocolate, sweet curd bars, jams).

- Canned food.

Substitute those with:

- Eggs, chicken, liver, fish, beans, cottage cheese.
- You can eat vegetables in any form, except canned. Eat sea kale.
- Spaghetti, brown rice, other pasta.
- Eat fruit in the morning. Grapes and bananas are excluded from this diet.
- Dried fruits - only 3 pieces a day. When buying dried fruits, be sure to check that there is no sugar.
- Honey - no more than 1 tsp per day.
- Nuts - 30-50 grams per day. Eat them raw.
- And drink lots of clean water!

The successful and healthy combination of protein, fats, and carbohydrates is:

30% protein, 10% fats, and 60% carbohydrates.

It will be hard, so hard for you to shift into a new diet! The body will require sweets, and at every step you will be stalked by sugar, sweets, and possible depression due to the absence of the usual set of goodies. Going to the store will be torture. It may even seem like there are almost no products that do not contain the harmful ingredient.

"For the sweet has to pay bitterly," - Leonardo da Vinci.

How do you turn white chocolate into dark chocolate?

Turn out the light.

You have to admit you are addicted! You are firmly hooked on the "white drug," which every day takes a big bite out of your health. And if you don't start fighting it right now, it is going to possess your future entirely. Appearance, health, psyche, tone, performance, and reproductive health will all be at risk!

Secret #7

Your sincere desire, patience, and willpower will help you overcome the sweets' abuse.

Chapter 4: Helpful Recipes

"Cooking is a pleasure, everyday, unfortunately,"
- American housewife

"A third of Americans want to lose weight, a third - to put it on,
and the other third has not yet been weighed,"
- John Steinbeck

What's a race car's favorite thing to eat for lunch?

Fast food!

Now, pay attention! This is what we call the climax. Here you'll find the most practical and result-oriented information for losing weight. In the previous chapters, we prepared you, motivated you, and set you up for victory over yourself and being overweight. The preparatory theoretical stage of mastering the 7 secrets is over. A positive personal example of the author convincingly proves that you can do it too! Put your hands on your belt and clasp your waist. Okay, now do you have the perfection to strive for? Making your waist thinner is real!

Practical cooking: Let's start with cooking food that helps lose and then maintain weight. We discussed breakfast in Chapter 3, but now we're moving on to lunch.

Lunch

"Ask not what you can do for your country. Ask what's for
lunch."
— Orson Welles

In my mind, the best meal is chicken, turkey, or low-fat beef with vegetables. It sounds ordinary, boring, and maybe even a bit prosaic, but a boiled fillet and a salad of Chinese cabbage immediately pop up before my eyes; something white, sooty, and tasteless, as if for babies or toothless elderly. But leave your panic, discouragement, and self-torture at the door! We are tuned in to the successful and interesting queen-worthy life. Therefore, the eating process is to be put on an appropriate level. Our dishes must satisfy, delight, and conform to the most exquisite tastes! (But don't forget about our goal to reduce ourselves in volume!)

There are many recipes for creating masterpieces out of these products.

- Meat and poultry can be baked in the oven until golden brown with various ingredients
- It can be cooked in foil, retaining amazing flavors
- It can be grilled, saturating the food with the energy of the open flame
- It can be turned into homemade sausages, twisted into small spirals
- It can be cut into delicious patties, steaks, chops, or schnitzels

We can change the shape of products, mince it, add spices and herbs... we have thousands of options, but we should do it without oil, or with a small amount of it.

"After a good dinner, one can forgive anybody, even one's own relations."
- Oscar Wilde, a Woman of No Importance

Scientists have found that the ordinary family has overall only 12 dishes on the menu, not more. But even this amount of change suits us! It is practical and fast, as family recipes emerge automatically.

Chicken in soy sauce and honey marinade

Ingredients:

- Chicken fillet - 1kg
- Soy sauce - 1 tablespoon (15g)
- Honey - 1 tablespoon (20g)
- Mustard (I take 1 teaspoon of ordinary strong mustard and 1 teaspoon of French mustard) - 1 tablespoon (15g)

- Olive oil - 1 tablespoon (15g)
- Garlic - 2-3 cloves (10g)
- Basil, parsley, paprika, black pepper, marjoram, dill
- Salt to taste

Preparation:

Prepare the marinade in a small deep bowl: mix soy sauce, honey, mustard, and olive oil. Salt the fillet, season it with spices, squeeze garlic, mix it with the fillet and put it into the prepared marinade. Cover and marinate overnight (but not less than 3 hours) in the fridge. In the morning, cook it! Take the baking pan, put some oil on it and lay out the marinated fillets. Put in an oven preheated to 180°C for about an hour or until done.

Homemade Turkey Sausages

Ingredients:

- Turkey fillet - 500 g
- Onions - 1 pcs
- Mustard (permitted for eating) -1 tsp
- Salt and pepper to taste

Preparation:

Cut the turkey fillet into pieces so that they fit into a blender or meat grinder. Add the onion. Then add salt, pepper, and season the meat with mustard. Process the mixture in a meat grinder or blender several times to make a gentle mince.

Cut the cling film into pieces and place the mince on them.

Tightly wrap it in plastic wrap, twist, and tie off both ends.

You can cook sausages immediately without removing the film. But to get a more elegant taste, cool the sausages in the fridge for 2 hours before cooking. Remove the film and then simmer them in boiling water or cook on the grill.

Chicken fillet skewers

Ingredients:

- Chicken fillet - 500 g
- Table vinegar - 40 ml
- Slices of garlic - 2 pcs
- Fresh ginger - 5 cm
- Soy sauce (without sugar) - 20 ml
- Green onions – 20 g
- Salt and pepper to taste

Preparation:

Peel the garlic and ginger, wash and dry the green onions.

Fold the spices into a blender and add vinegar and soy sauce. Beat until smooth. Peel the fillets and cut them into small pieces (4-5 cm). Put the meat into the bag with the marinade, add salt and pepper, close tightly, and distribute the marinade so that it covers the meat from all sides. Leave the meat-marinade mixture in the refrigerator for several hours. String marinated pieces on long wooden skewers and put them on a preheated grill pan. Fry and turn the meat so that it is evenly roasted on all sides and cooked thoroughly.

Turkey rolls with greens

Ingredients:

- Turkey breast - 800 g
- Greens - 1 bunch (to your taste)
- Black pepper and salt - to taste

Preparation:

Spread the skinless turkey fillet and lightly beat it to a thickness of 0.5 cm. Add salt and pepper. For the stuffing, put the washed greens into the blender. Add salt and pepper. Grind until you get the mashed potatoes texture. Spread the breast and stuff it with ground greens. Carefully roll up the breasts and tightly wrap in a plastic wrap like a candy. Twist the ends. In a deep saucepan, boil salted water. Put the turkey rolls in and cook them for 20 minutes on medium heat. Remove the roll from the boiling water with a skimmer, allow it cool slightly and remove the film. Cut into small pieces.

Juicy beef patties

Ingredients:

- Beef mince - 400g
- Carrots -2pcs
- Zucchini (squash) -2pc
- Eggs - 2pcs
- Onions - 1 pc
- Spices to taste
- You can add any of your favorite vegetables.

Preparation:

Shred carrots, zucchini and onions, mix them with minced meat, eggs, and spices. Form the cutlets with wet hands and bake them in the oven at 180°C until golden brown (20-40 minutes depending on the size).

Chicken with vegetables

Ingredients:
- Fillet - 800 g
- White mushrooms - 250-300 g
- Bell pepper - 2 pcs
- Onion - 1 pc
- Carrots - 1 pc
- Tomato paste - 1 tbsp
- Some fresh dill
- Salt and pepper to taste

Preparation:

Cut the chicken fillet into small pieces and fry using minimum oil. Add chopped onion half-rings to the meat, and mix and fry for another 3 minutes. Put in the pepper and halved mushrooms. If the mushrooms are large, then cut them into quarters. In case they are small, don't cut them at all. Add shredded carrots and tomato paste and fry for another 5 minutes. Then pour 300 ml of water and simmer on low for about 30 minutes. Stir a couple of times, while simmering, and add water if necessary.

Zucchini Ragout with Tomatoes and Garlic

Ingredients:
- Zucchini - 2 kg
- Tomato - 500 g
- 1 garlic clove
- Bunch of Parsley
- Salt, ground pepper - to taste
- Dried herbs, better ready mix: Italian or Provencal herbs to taste.

Preparation:

Clear the tails off the zucchini, cut into cubes. Finely chop the onion, and cut tomatoes into cubes as well. On high, fry the onions until soft. Add zucchini and fry until golden. Next, put in the tomatoes and mix. Stew on high heat for a few minutes, then, add salt and pepper. Add dried herbs and squeeze in the garlic.

Stir and continue to simmer, trying not to turn the contents into squash paste. Meanwhile, finely chop the parsley and serve ragout sprinkled with herbs. The dish is equally good hot or cold. You can sprinkle the stew with cheese and put it in the oven for 5 minutes.

We're going to end the chapter on cooking with dinner recommendations.

Hope is a good breakfast, but a poor supper.

To feed yourself, not only with hopes for weight loss, dinner must be within reasonable limits and of a special quality.

Stewed vegetables, all kinds of soups, or vegetable casseroles decorated with a piece of lean chicken, fish, or cottage cheese of choice. In the evening, your body also needs protein, but stew vegetables, so that the body does not get agitated before going to bed with raw vegetables. Abandon pastries and potatoes for dinner.

A man ordered a takeout pizza. The waiter said: "Shall I cut it into six pieces or twelve?"

"Six, please. I could never eat twelve."

Click http://e-book.tilda.ws/rideawave2 and you will get another 20 receipts from me! It`s my gift for you!

Chapter 5: Training and Problem Areas

"With the help of physical exercises and self-control, most people can do without medicine." - Joseph Addison

"Nothing depletes and destroys the human body as physical inactivity." - Aristotle

A healthy body is:

- flexible, pliable, elastic
- strong, solid, enduring
- harmonic, proportional, balanced

The better a person owns their body, the better he or she will manage life and the more easy-going they are when communicating with others.

The body's systems must also meet the following "standards":

- ✓ muscles and bands are toned
- ✓ joints are movable and flexible
- ✓ spine cord is straight, flexible, easily curled
- ✓ core helps maintain posture
- ✓ neck is flexible, head is raised high,
- ✓ face is relaxed, has an slightly open smile
- ✓ the stomach is strapped, the waist is thin
- ✓ thighs, legs, and buttocks are elastic, pumped up
- ✓ the feet are springy, and no flat feet
- ✓ blood is saturated, hemoglobin level is fine
- ✓ all natural physiological processes are normal

Health is maintained with a set of activities, one of which is exercising.

We're not going to give you the well-known basic exercises that you can learn to do in any gym, as you can learn that anywhere.

Instead, we're going to concentrate on problem areas: the abdomen, waist, hips, buttocks, and back.

Anecdote
Why do hamburgers go to the gym? To get better buns!

Important!

We're always taking into account the preparedness, health condition, individual characteristics, age, instructions of specialists, and personal preferences.

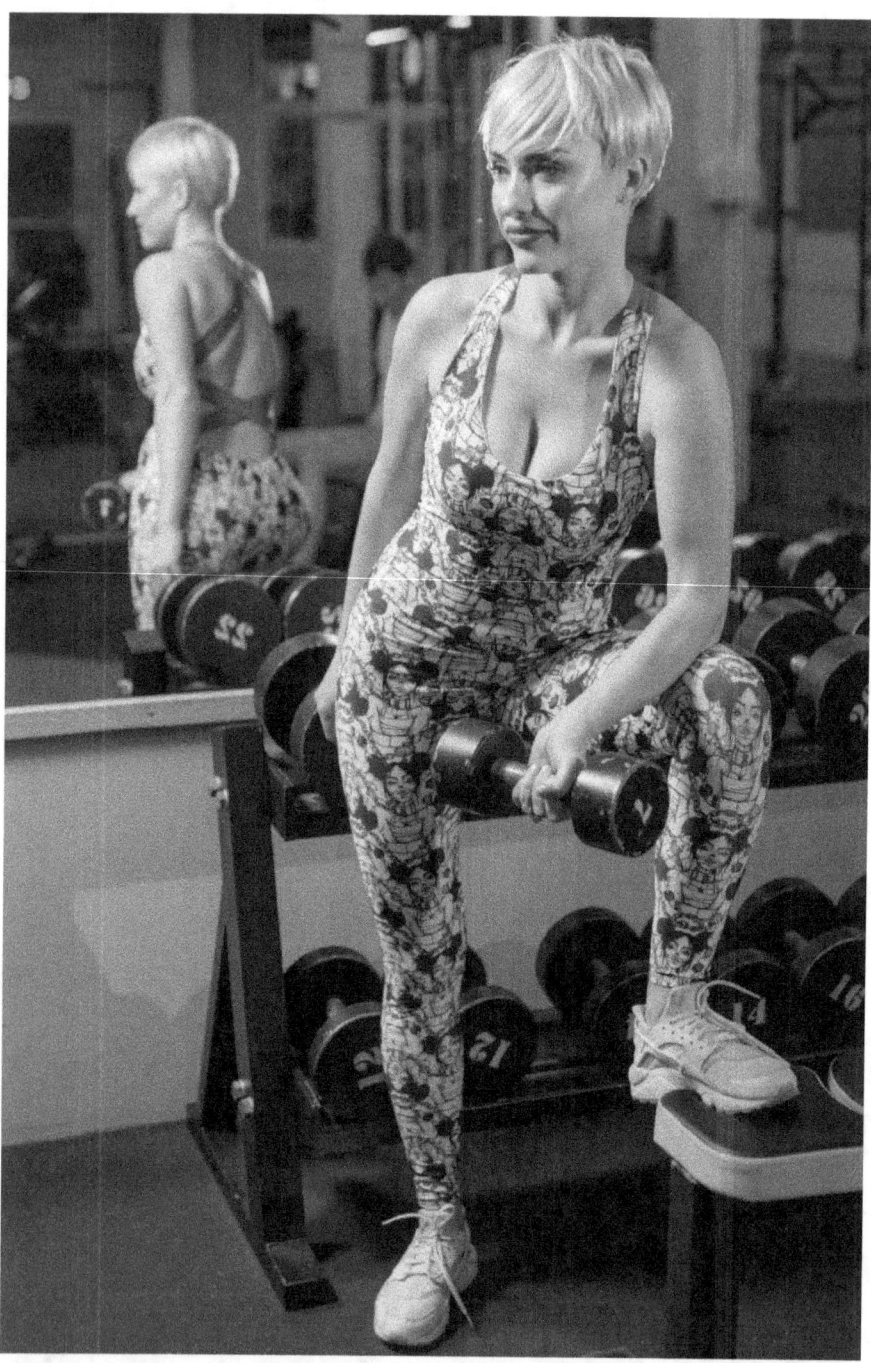

An exercise set should include the many factors that you must discuss with professional trainers. If you have any chronic disease or any other health problem, it is important to consult with a reflex therapist, a rehabilitation specialist, or a physiotherapist. And some might even need guidance from an allergist, an immunologist, or another specialist.

First, diagnose and audit your own body, find out whether your body works well as a system; examine and test your health. It may appear that you lack the vitamins and minerals needed for having a normal life in general.

Create a diary and write the initial weight you had at the start of the weight loss plan. Remember, of course, the goal is the weight desired in specific numbers. Be sure to take a photo for future comparison at the beginning of this journey. And don't forget to make regular records of your achievements.

Be sure to work on the machines.

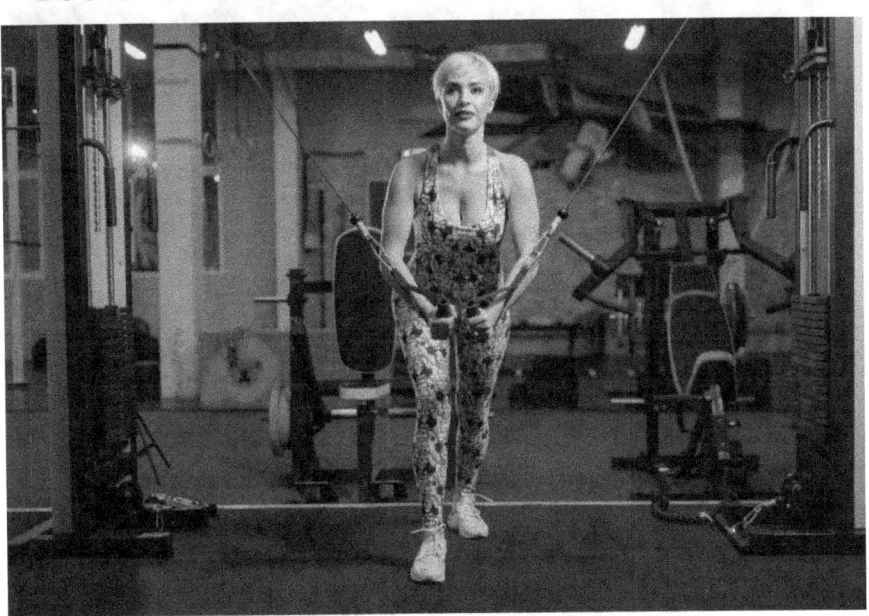

First, choose the appropriate training plan.

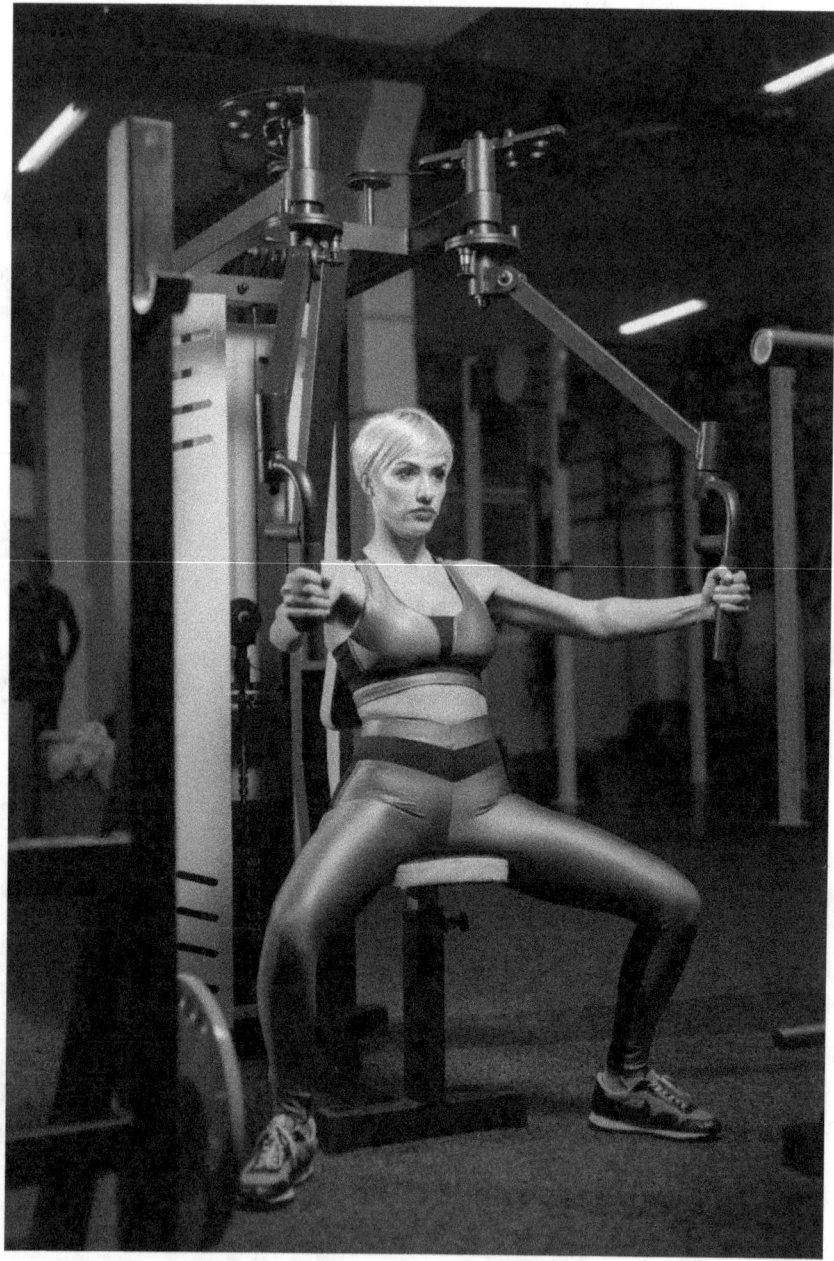

Problem areas: abdomen, buttocks, thighs, and back.

Now go directly to exercising. Here are **5 exercises for the hips and buttocks.**

5 Exercices Efficaces Qui Vont Développer Vos Fessiers & Améliorer Votre Posture

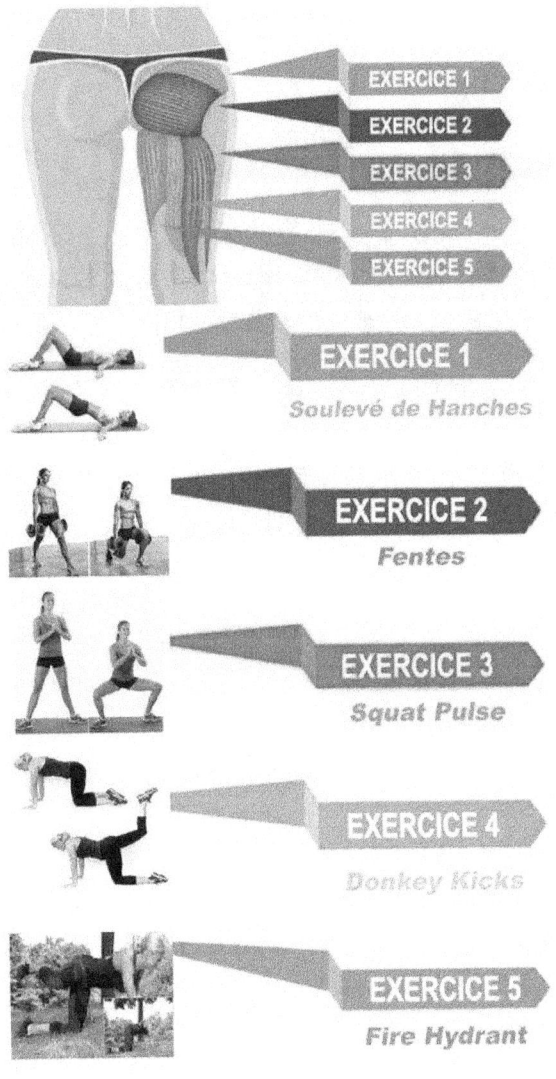

EXERCICE 1

EXERCICE 2

EXERCICE 3

EXERCICE 4

EXERCICE 5

EXERCICE 1
Soulevé de Hanches

EXERCICE 2
Fentes

EXERCICE 3
Squat Pulse

EXERCICE 4
Donkey Kicks

EXERCICE 5
Fire Hydrant

1. Glute Bridge

Do it after the basic exercises. Lie on your back on the mat and stretch your arms along the body, palms down. Bend your legs at the knees. Put your tightened feet as close to the buttocks as you can. Feet and knees should be hip width. The body and hands are tightly pressed to the floor. Technique: you cannot tear off the shoulders and stand up on the back of your head. Raise the hips! The upper torso, head, and arms remain motionless on the floor! We will focus on the muscles, linger for 1-2 seconds, and put the hips down. There should be 3 sets of 10-20 reps.

2. Lunges

Lunges are the most effective strength exercises for the buttocks and thigh muscles. You can do lunges forward, backward, sideways, and diagonally, with or without extra weight. There are about 20 modifications. With a set of lunges, you can achieve impressive results. We will first master the technique without additional weight, but we will gradually increase the load.

The classic way: Stand up straight, with legs slightly apart so that the foot, knee, thigh, and shoulders form a straight line. While inhaling, take a step forward and shift the weight to the front foot. The hips and legs should make a right angle. On the exhale, push the heel off from the floor, tighten the muscles of the buttocks and the back of the thigh, and return to the starting position. There should be 3 sets of 10 for each leg.

3. Wide-feet squats, Sumo squats

First, you need to stand up straight and get into a natural position in the back. The legs are to the sides and your feet are turned to the outside. The width between your legs and the turning angle should be chosen individually, but you should try to place the legs as wide as possible and rotate them to 45 degrees. First, practice squatting several times without weight. If you manage to bring your hips in parallel with the floor and, at the same time you don't feel any imposition, continue doing the exercise in this position. Exercise is performed in 3-4 sets with 10-15 reps.

4. Donkey Kicks (raising the leg up while standing on the knees).

Initial position - the emphasis is on the knee, the bent right leg is raised up. The hip is parallel to the floor, the angle at the knee is about 90 degrees, and the foot is turned to the ceiling. Hold the leg in this position for 10-60 seconds. Then do springing movements with leg up to 20-30cm, having the thigh in parallel with the floor, but not lowered. The angle in the knee remains unchanged and the foot "pushes" towards the ceiling. Repeat 10-50 times.

5. Fire hydrant (lifting the bent leg to the side while standing on the knees and hands). Both legs are bent at 90°. Repeat 10-50 times.

Before doing the exercises, be sure to knock-up, warm up, and set the base. Want to only do these exercises? Run for 4-5 minutes.

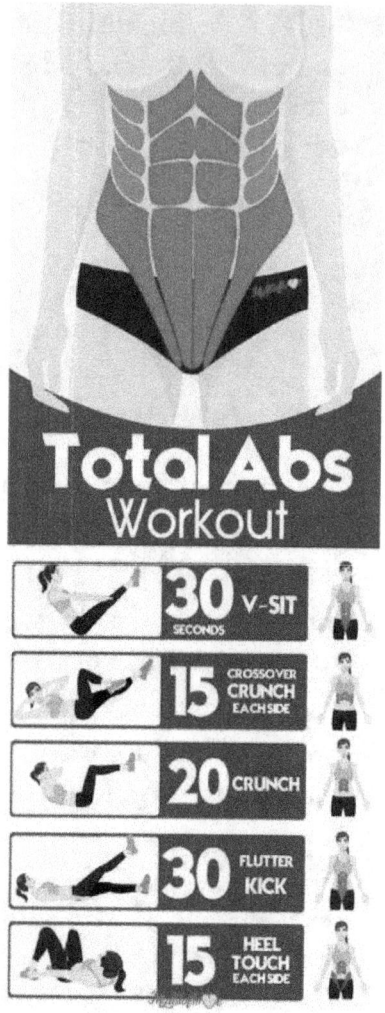

1. V-sit - Sitting on the floor, raise your legs by 45°. Hold for 30 seconds.

2. Bicycle - As in the previous exercise, put your hands behind your head, bend one leg, and leave the other straight. Twist the torso, pulling the elbows to the knees. There should be15 twists.

3. Crunches or twisting turns - Put your legs on a stand to make a 90° angle. Put your hands behind your head. Let there be 20 reps.

4. Walk your legs up and down, lying on your backs. Let there be 30 reps.

5. While lying on your back, set your feet and thighs wide with legs bent at the knees. Stretch a hand out to one leg, then to the other, bending to the side of the waist and trying to touch your heels. There should be 15 touches in both directions.

To make the back and the whole body strong, use the **plank position.**

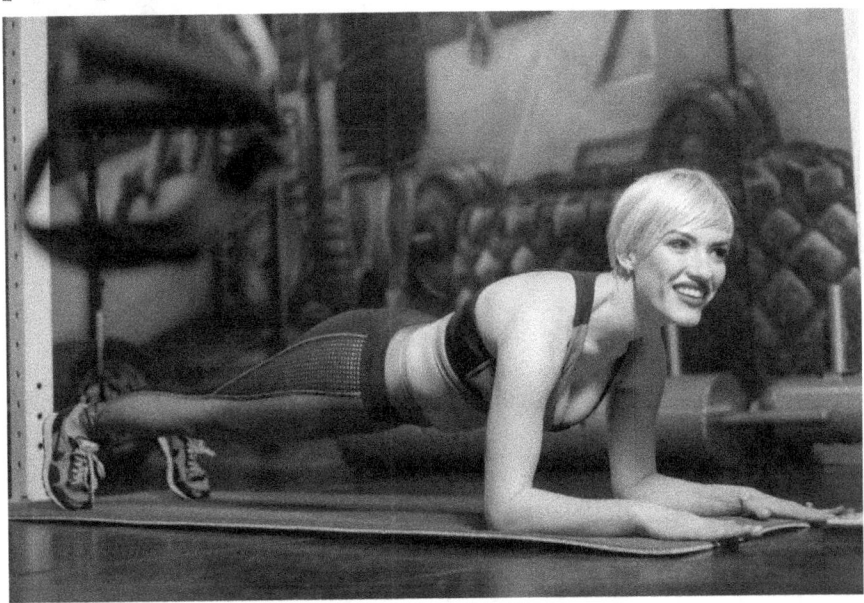

My fitness coach told me to bend down and touch my toes. I said, "I don't have that kind of relationship with my feet. Can I just wave?"

Our task is to tighten the whole body, to force ourselves to be engaged not only with the physical indicators - weight and volume. We must also train qualities of character; for example, perseverance, endurance, and consistency.

We keep a diary, record the results, team up with others and share our achievements. During the training, don't forget to smile.

Exercising with a high weight without conscious work on yourself, won't bring anything!

You are not a machine gun; you don't have to train with the autopilot on. Pay attention to yourself, the responses and reactions of your body, and any gratitude or pleasure from the process. They train your overall character and willpower.

Introduce competition into the weight reduction process – in other words, overcome challenges daily both yours and of those who train next to you.

Chapter 6: Secrets, Clues, and Vital Things

"Compare your desires with the ones of others and make conclusions – it is a simple way of studying in this world." - Hong Zicheng

"Change begets change." - Charles Dickens

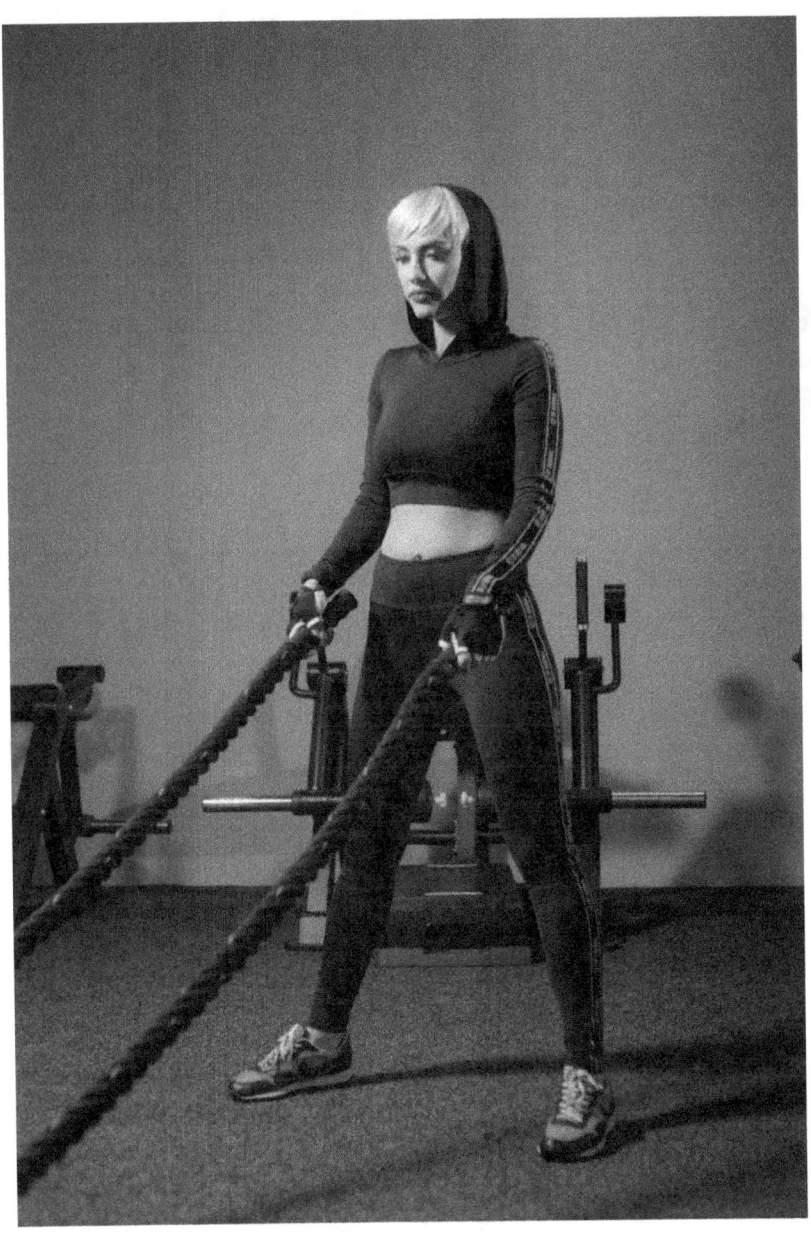

This is the chapter where all of the highlights from the rest of the book are gathered. We figured out why you need to lose weight and the personal reason has been recognized. To firmly walk forward onto the path of weight loss, we must also recognize the advantages of a sporting figure:

- a gorgeous and sexy appearance;
- excellent health;
- self-confidence;
- career advancement;
- can fit in new trendy clothes and bikinis;
- the prospect of having easier relationships and a long-lasting life.

Future positive changes lead to the restoration of the body's self-regulatory processes, the gaining of willpower, and the overcoming of food dependence.

After reading this book, you can come to these conclusions:

- The only way to lose weight is to redefine your goals in life. What are your priorities? Is what is on the outside reflective of what's on the inside?
- The habit of eating moderately is one that distances oneself from the acute problems of the self. A person who found his place and eats for life, but not lives for eating, spends his power on the most important things in life.
- Homemade food is the happiest food for the family. It unites, strengthens family ties, and it reinforces family traditions. Cooking at home is self-love and self-care!
- Pay attention to the food that your children eat at school. Perhaps pack a lunch for them that you think is healthier.
- Explain to your relatives about how to keep track of their weight and how to take care of themselves. Do

not put the attainment of this important skill on the shoulders of the education and healthcare systems.

- Not all adolescent problems can be attributed to this transitional age. Paying attention to their psychological needs will reduce or discourage consumption of sweets, as it is being substituted by real-life human communication.

- Following yourself and family to control the food is not becoming a bad habit. Constantly pay attention to what you buy at the store. Apply critical thinking to the 12 common dishes you cook for your family. Is it time to reconsider the usual diet and move in the direction of positive change?

- Is the gym comfortable for you psychologically? Perhaps you need to change the coach or choose one that is more suitable for women. Today, there's a huge variety of possible options -aerobics of several types: step, aqua, jazz, yoga, cycling aerobics, aerobics with a skipping rope, fit ball exercises. There are lots of other traditional and new types of training systems as well, such as yoga, callanetics, strip-dance, body flex, shaping, spinning, cycling, resist-a-ball, pole-dance, Body Ballet, Nordic walking, hooping, stiletto, etc.

- While working in the gym, pay attention to the rules and established traditions. Watch others and be polite and respectful. Put the inventory back where you found it.

- Help other people who are overweight. Protect them from bullying during their workouts, support them psychologically, and cheer them up.

- Get rid of baking sweets as a hobby! Find something else, maybe something better suited for the athletic type.

- If someone else in your family wants to lose weight, support them with faith and encouragement. Treat intentions to change with respect.
- At work, do not talk about your efforts to lose weight. There will always be evil tongues and provocateurs. Personal business is not for public display.
- Work is important. But don't get too attached; don't stick to it with your whole being. Stress is due to the great dependence on the results. Treat your achievements with a small amount of humor.
- Don't call yourself offensive nicknames. The subconscious mind records everything. It will be difficult to uproot these weeds, so it's better to praise yourself, even for the small victories.
- Make a picture and film in your mind of a perfect version of yourself in detail. Play this movie continuously. The work of thought is more important than anything else!
- Stop eating junk food, sweets, and other harmful products. Resist temptation! What we do need is to refresh the consciousness regularly! Experience and feel something new from time to time.
- Find a suitable recovery system that meets your needs and wishes, and stick to it.. Do not change the selected path. You may adjust the details, but the overall path must remain unchanged.
- Choose a diet. We recommend eating five different fruits and veggies daily. Include a variety of colors in your produce and make an effort into how you serve your food.
- Study books and films about a healthy lifestyle and share knowledge with friends and family. Be sure to have a strong desire, and iron will, and monk-like patience. These qualities will definitely help you overcome not only the excess weight but also other

difficulties that may happen in your life. Stop expecting instant results! Lasting changes require time and effort!

Summary

1. Scientists have proven that after reading a book once, a person learns 20% of what they read. Therefore, in order to get the full 100% result, read the data four more times.

2. Introduce innovations in small steps. Start change with tiny steps. The overall effect is going to be impressive.

3. Practice and action lead to the desired reflection in the mirror. Reading alone is not enough.

4. Each chapter carries interesting and useful secrets; together, the book turns out to be a system of guidance based on the real-life story of the author.

5. It doesn't matter where you start! Just take the first step. Then one more. Then another. And then another.

6. Praise yourself for any victory over yourself, even when you think it's nothing. The subconscious will quickly get used to "the winner" psychology.

7. Penalize yourself with money for missing training sessions or breaking your diet and routine.

8. Promise yourself a prize in writing at the end of the training phase and after achieving a winning weight.

9. Lose weight only for your own sake, not for anyone else's. Do it for healing, rejuvenation, and to improve the quality of your life.

10. Compete! Make losing weight an adventure. Let the tinge of a fun game be present when training! More jokes, more humor!

11. Whenever you fall off the horse, get back on and try again!

12. Ride the wave! You CAN do it!

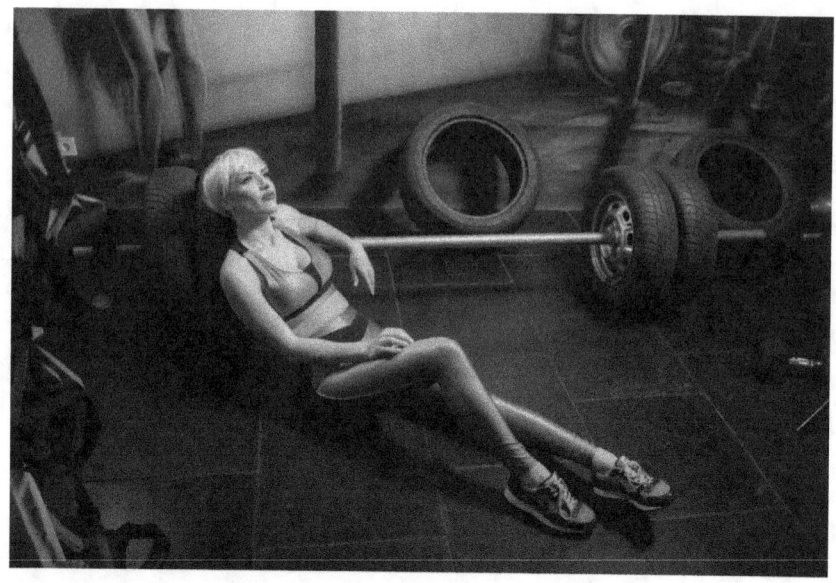

"Eighty percent of success is showing up." – Woody Allen

"The only beauty I know is health." - Heinrich Heine

"Life is the path, the goal and the reward. Life is a dance of love. Your mission is to bloom. BEING is a great gift to the world. Your life is the story of the Universe. That's why life is more beautiful than all the theories." - King Solomon

Thank you for reading my book! If you want to contact me or to ask any questions, please right me on email: anastasia.turner2019@gmail.com and of course you can leave me a feedback about my book!

www.ingramcontent.com/pod-product-compliance
Lightning Source LLC
Chambersburg PA
CBHW072121280526
45788CB00006B/2578